The Sheep Brain: A Basic Guide

Richard K. Cooley and C.H. Vanderwolf

A.J. Kirby Co.
London, Ontario, Canada

ISBN: 0920700012

A.J. Kirby Co.
London, Ontario, Canada

www.ajkirbyco.com

Printed in Canada

Introduction

In the beginning of the 21th century, we appear to be in the midst of a period of spectacular advance in our understanding of the nervous system and the way it works to generate behavior. The advances in scientific knowledge have made possible great improvements in the medical treatment of a number of neurological and psychiatric disorders in man. It is reasonable to expect even greater successes in the future as scientific knowledge increases.

This little book is intended as an elementary introduction to the structure and function of the nervous system. The sheep brain is recommended as material for study since it is a convenient size and is readily available at low cost from butchers or from biological supply houses.

In the pages to follow the authors have prepared various labeled views of the sheep brain. Explanatory text accompanies each photograph.

R.K.C
C.H.V.

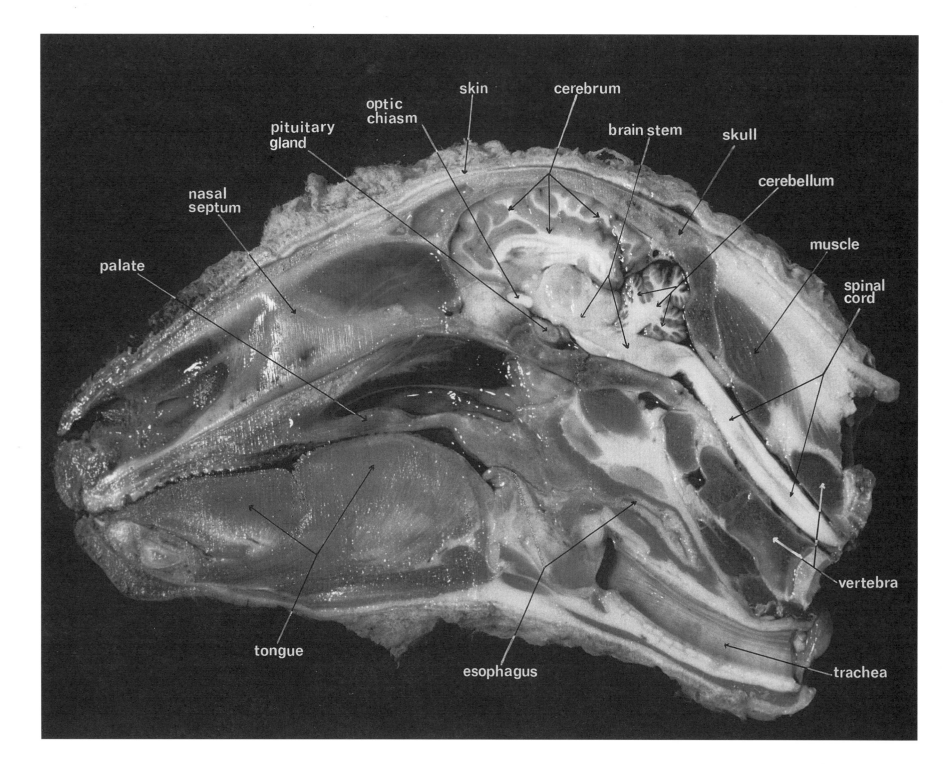

Figure 1. The brain in relation to the other structures of the head.

This photograph was prepared from the right half of the head of a freshly slaughtered lamb which was frozen and cut into two longitudinal halves with a band saw. The cut was made slightly to the left of the midline (an imaginary plane dividing the body into equal right and left halves). Note how the spinal cord lies enclosed in a bony tube formed by the successive vertebrae. It passes into the skull via the foramen magnum (Latin: big hole) where it is continuous with the medulla (also known as the medulla oblongata or the bulb). The medulla, pons, and midbrain (see Figures 5,6, & 7) together constitute the brainstem. Sometimes the thalamus and hypothalamus (Figure 6) are also considered as part of the brainstem. Attached to the base of the hypothalamus is the pituitary gland, an endocrine gland of great importance in development and the regulation of a variety of body processes.

The brain and spinal cord are protected from direct contact with the bony skull and vertebral column by enclosure in a tough skin-like bag, the dura mater or dura. Inside the dura are thinner membranes, one of which, the pia mater or pia, is closely adherent to the nervous tissue itself. A third membrane, the arachnoid, lies between the pia and dura and is loosely attached to them, particularly to the pia. The three membranes together are known as the meninges. The spaces between the meninges, particularly the one between the pia and the arachnoid, are filled during life with a colorless watery fluid known as the cerebrospinal fluid. The meninges and the cerebrospinal fluid protect the brain from vibration or sudden jarring as would be encountered in running, jumping or blows to the head.

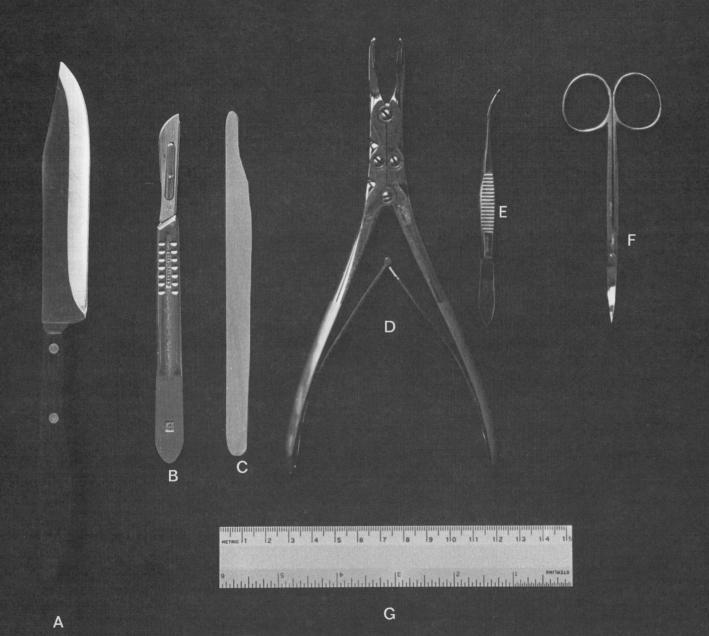

A

B

C

D

E

F

METRIC 1 2 3 4 5 6 7 8 9 10 11 12 13 14 15

G

Figure 2. Methods for the study of the sheep brain.

The sheep brains available from biological supply houses are usually provided with the skull and part of the dura already removed. Simple dissecting instruments, of the type shown here, are adequate for a gross examination of the brain.

If you choose to work with a complete sheep head (either fresh or preserved) begin by removing any vertebrae that may be attached to the skull and remove the skin and muscle from the top and sides of the head. This can be done with a scalpel (B). Then, using the rongeurs (D) or an autopsy saw (if available) remove the top and sides of the skull. A convenient place to begin this procedure is provided by the foramen magnum, the hole through which the spinal cord leaves the skull (Figure 1). Try to avoid damaging the dura as you remove the skull. In places where the dura adheres tightly to the skull separate the two with a thin <u>blunt</u> instrument, such as a thin flat piece of wood (C). When the brain, still enclosed in the dura, is fully exposed raise it very gently and cut the cranial nerves (see Figure 5) as close to the skull as possible.

A fresh brain can be preserved and hardened by placing it in a solution of formaldehyde. Formaldehyde (H_2CO) is a noxious gas available (at hardware, agricultural or scientific supply stores) as a solution in water. This solution (formalin) should be diluted to 10% for use as a preservative. If table salt (NaCL) is added to make a 0.9% solution it will prevent the brain from absorbing water and swelling slightly. To make one liter of solution, containing 10% formalin (by volume) and 0.9% NaCL (by weight) add 9 gms of NaCL to 100 mls of formalin. Then add enough water to make exactly one liter. Stir until the NaCL is fully dissolved.

Before immersing a fresh brain in a formalin solution make several cuts in the dura, using the scissors (F) to allow the solution ready access to the brain.

When the brain has been allowed to harden in the formalin solution for several days it is ready for examination. Remove the dura using forceps and scissors. Since formalin will "preserve" human skin as well as sheep brain it is advisable to wear rubber gloves when handling formalin treated material. If formalin is accidentally splashed in the eyes, rinse immediately with large quantities of clean water.

The following pages illustrate some of the features of a sheep brain. During dissection a sharp knife with a thin blade (A) can be used to cut the brain into sections but a smaller scalped (B) is better for trimming or slicing off smaller pieces. A blunt edged wooden stick (C) made from some sort of soft wood is better than a steel knife for scraping away tissue. Such a stick can be made from coffee stirrers, tongue depressors, etc. The small forceps (E) and scissors (F) are useful for removing the meninges surrounding the brain, cutting cranial nerves, etc.

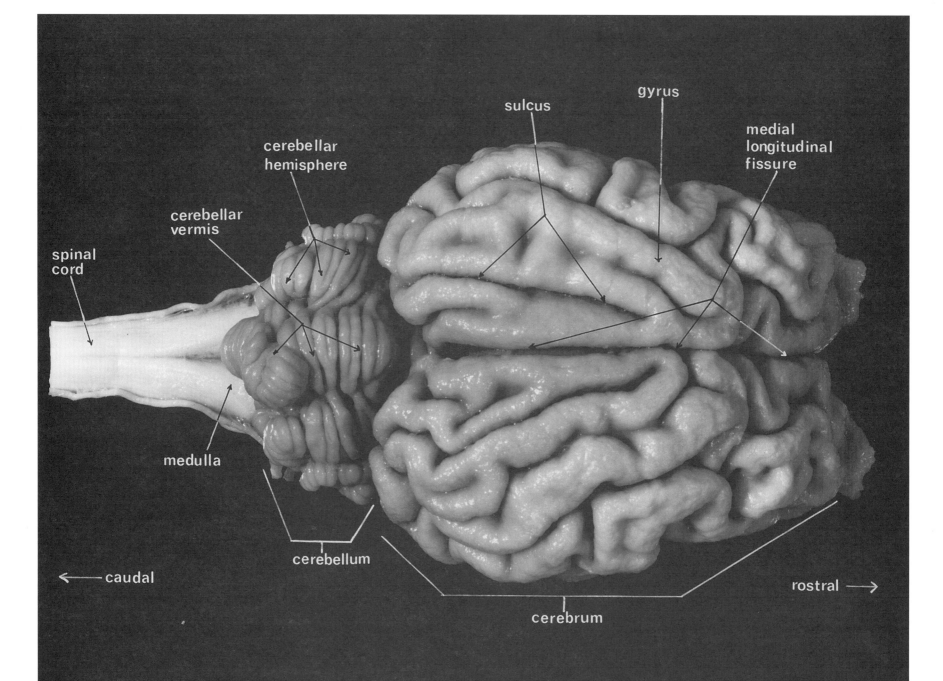

sulcus

gyrus

medial longitudinal fissure

cerebellar hemisphere

cerebellar vermis

spinal cord

medulla

cerebellum

caudal

rostral

cerebrum

Figure 3. Dorsal view of a sheep brain.

The various possible views of an anatomical structure are referred to as dorsal (Latin: dorsum = back) for a top view; ventral (Latin: venter = belly) for a view from the underside; rostral (Latin: rostrum = beak) for a front view; caudal (Latin: cauda = tail) for a rear view; lateral for a side view and medial for a view from the midline. The same terms are applied to regions within a structure, e.g. the medial hypothalamus, or the caudal part of the midbrain.

Note the gross divisions of the brain which are visible in a dorsal view. The brainstem is completely covered by the cerebellum and cerebrum except for the caudal part of the medulla. The cerebellum consists of a medially placed vermis (It looks a bit like a worm. Latin: vermis = worm) and two laterally placed hemispheres. The entire outer surface of the cerebellum consists of the cerebellar cortex (Latin: cortex = bark) which is folded up into a series of narrow ridges called folia (singular, folium).

The cerebrum is divided into left and right halves, the cerebral hemispheres, by the medial longitudinal fissure. As in the cerebellum, the outer surface consists of cortex, the cerebral cortex, folded into a series of ridges. In the cerebrum, these ridges are called gyri (singular, gyrus) and the furrows separating them are called either sulci (singular, sulcus) or fissures. The sulci are filled with many small blood vessels and with the pia and arachnoid membranes. If these are pulled out carefully with fine forceps the depths of the sulci can be seen. If the cerebral hemispheres are spread slightly and the blood vessels and pia are removed, it is possible to see a heavy band of white fibres connecting the hemispheres. This is the corpus callosum.

Gently spread apart the cerebellum and the cerebrum. Pick out the pia and blood vessels to expose four rounded mounds, the superior and inferior colliculi (see Figure 7). In sheep, the superior colliculi are much larger and better developed than the inferior colliculi.

When examining the brain notice that some structures (the optic nerves are a good example) are glistening white while others are of a dull grey or ivory color (the cortex is a good example). These color differences are the basis of the terms "grey matter" and "white matter". White matter owes its color to the presence of large numbers of myelinated (myelin covered) nerve fibres while grey matter consists of nerve cell bodies and fine unmyelinated fibres.

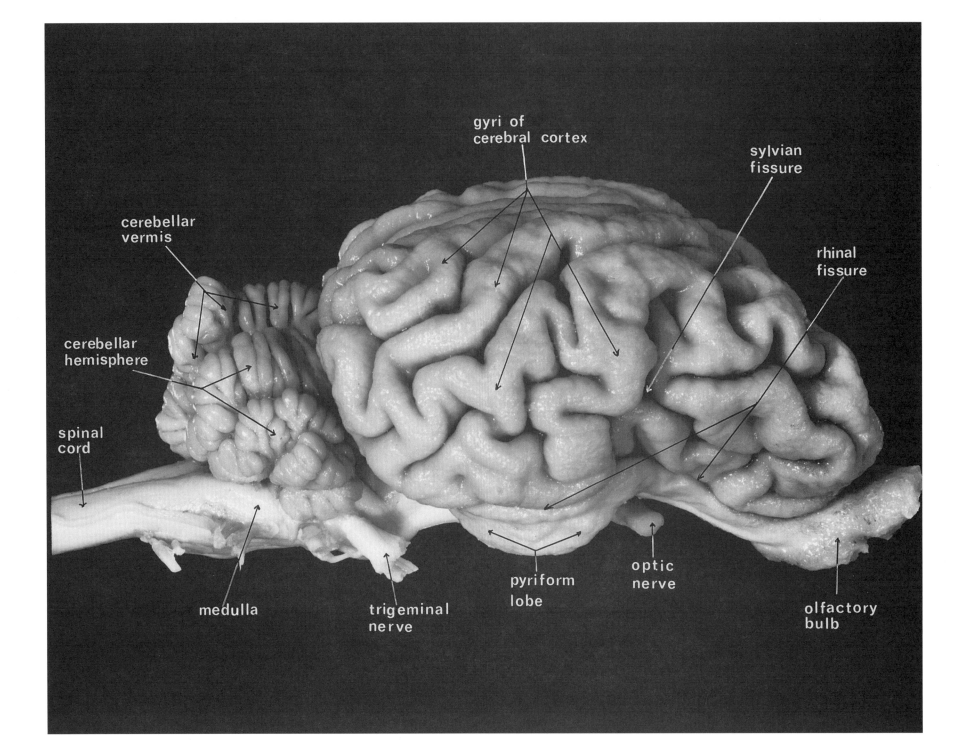

Figure 4. Lateral view of a sheep brain.

Many of the structures visible in a dorsal view can also be seen from the side. A number of cranial nerves (trigeminal nerve, optic nerve) can be seen, and the side of the brainstem is partly visible.

The fissures and sulci of the cerebral cortex are quite variable from one species of animal to another. However, one fissure, the rhinal fissure, is present in nearly all mammals, including man. This fissure is the dividing line between the pyriform lobe, located ventrally, and the neocortex which is the prominent furrowed type of cerebral cortex visible in dorso-lateral views of the brain. Thus the cerebral cortex as a whole includes the hippocampal formation (see Figure 7) and the medial strip of cortex lying immediately dorsal to the corpus callosum.

The subdivisions of the cerebral cortex are developed to different degrees in different kinds of animals. For example, something resembling the pyriform lobe can be recognized in various kinds of amphibia, fish and reptiles but none of these animals has a tissue that closely resembles the neocortex. This fact suggests that some of the differences in behavior between mammals and other animals may depend on the presence of the neocortex.

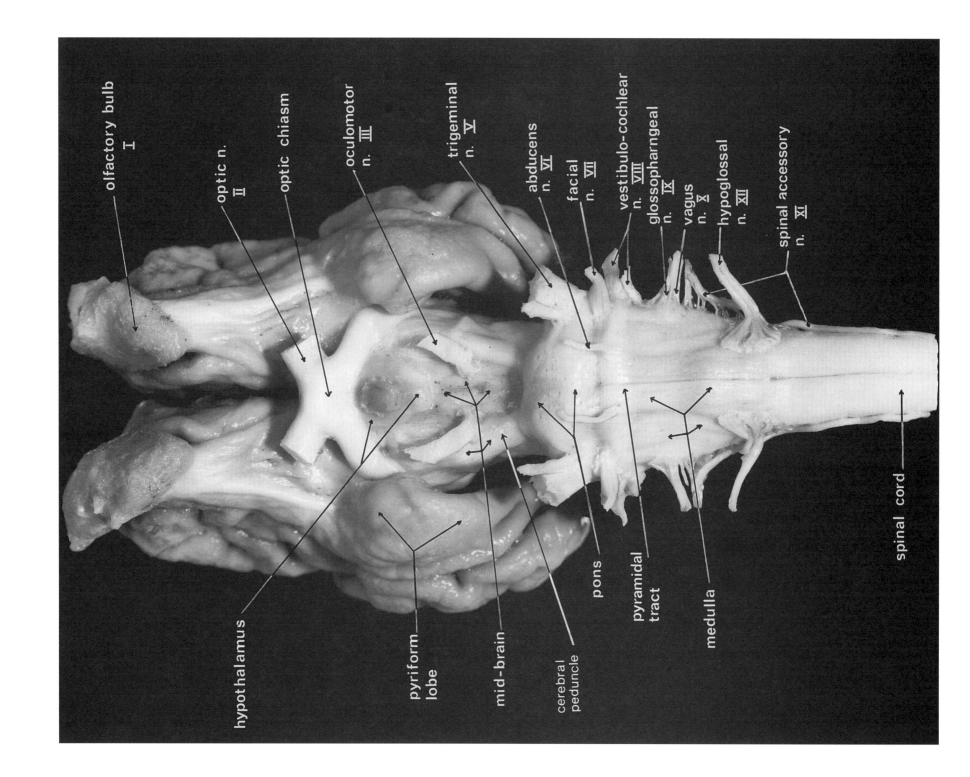

olfactory bulb I

optic n. II

optic chiasm

oculomotor n. III

trigeminal n. V

abducens n. VI

facial n. VII

vestibulo-cochlear n. VIII

glossopharngeal n. IX

vagus n. X

hypoglossal n. XII

spinal accessory n. XI

hypothalamus

pyriform lobe

mid-brain

cerebral peduncle

pons

pyramidal tract

medulla

spinal cord

Figure 5. Ventral view of a sheep brain.

A ventral view reveals the underside of the brainstem and nearly all the cranial nerves as well as the pyriform lobe. In this photograph, the pituitary gland has been removed to reveal the hypothalamus. Note that the floor of the midbrain consists of the two cerebral peduncles (Latin: pedunculus = stem) separated by an interpeduncular space. These peduncles disappear under the surface of the pons (Latin: pontis = bridge) but some of the fibres which they contain re-emerge as the pyramidal tracts which appear on the medial surface of the medulla. Axons which run in the pyramidal tracts originate mainly from cells in the rostral neocortex, run successively through the corona radiata and internal capsule (see page 19), then through the cerebral peduncle and pyramidal tract before finally terminating in the spinal cord. In the medulla, just above the spinal cord, many of the axons of these corticospinal neurons cross to the opposite side of the nervous system. That is, axons from the left cortex run mainly to the right side of the spinal cord while axons from the right cortex run mainly to the left side of the spinal cord. Corticospinal cells play a role in the control of movement, permitting the neocortex of each cerebral hemisphere to exert a direct effect on the activity of spinal neurons which run to muscles on the opposite side of the body.

Mammals have twelve pairs of cranial nerves which are referred to by English or Latin names and also by numbers, beginning at the rostral end of the brain.

I   Olfactory Nerve

The first cranial nerve or olfactory nerve is a sensory nerve consisting of thin fibres running from the olfactory mucosa (a patch of odor-sensitive tissue high up in the nasal sinuses) to the olfactory bulb. These fine fibres are always torn off when the brain is removed from the skull. Destruction of the olfactory mucosa, the nerve fibres or the olfactory bulbs results in anosmia, an inability to detect odors.

II   Optic Nerve

The optic nerve is a sensory nerve which carries information about the visual world from the eye to the brain. The retina in the eye contains specialized receptor cells which react to light. These cells act on other cells through several synapses, finally exciting the retinal ganglion cells whose axons leave the eye in the optic nerve. The optic nerves form a chiasma (Greek: chiasma = cross) at the base of the brain. In the optic chiasma some of the fibres from the left eye cross to the right side of the brain and some of the fibres do not cross in this way. Similarly, some of the fibres from the right eye cross to the left side of the brain. As a result of this incomplete crossing, the optic nerve caudal to the chiasma (it is called the optic tract caudal to the chiasma), contains fibres from both eyes. Damage to the optic tract, therefore, will produce partial blindness in both eyes while damage to the optic nerve fibres between the retina and the optic chiasma will produce blindness in one eye only.

11

III   Oculomotor Nerve

The oculomotor nerve is a motor nerve some of whose fibres control the activity of muscles that turn the eyeball in its socket (extraocular muscles). Action potentials passing outward in others of the fibres of the third nerve cause (via a synapse and a second neuron) the pupil of the eye to constrict. This happens whenever the eye is exposed to a bright light. Fibres of the oculomotor nerve also control a tiny muscle which changes the shape of the lens in order to focus sharply the images of objects located at various distances from the eye.

IV   Trochlear Nerve

The trochlear nerve shares with the oculomotor and abducens nerves the function of controlling the extraocular muscles. It is not visible on the ventral surface of the brain but can be found emerging just behind the inferior colliculus.

V   Trigeminal Nerve

The trigeminal nerve (tri + Latin: geminus = twin) is a mixed nerve which means that it contains both sensory and motor fibres. The main portion, which is split into three divisions, carries sensory information from the skin, muscles and other structures of the head such as the bones and teeth. A dentist can reduce or abolish the pain produced by drilling in teeth by injecting a local anesthetic into the vicinity of branches of the Vth nerve. Local anesthetics are drugs that block the passage of nerve impulses. After injection, drilling can still set up nerve impulses at the ends of the nerve fibres but because these impulses cannot reach the brain, no pain is felt.

In addition to the sensory branches the trigeminal nerve includes a motor nerve which runs to the jaw muscles to control biting and chewing.

VI   Abducens

The abducens is a pure motor nerve which together with the oculomotor and trochlear nerves, controls, the movements of the eye.

VII   Facial

The facial nerve is a mixed nerve, carrying sensory fibres for taste from the tongue as well as motor fibres to the muscles of the face. Movements such as winking or smiling depend upon an intact facial nerve. Other motor fibres run to the salivary glands and tear glands to produce, respectively, salivation and the secretion of tears.

VIII   Vestibulo-cochlear Nerve

The VIIIth nerve is a sensory nerve consisting of a cochlear division and a vestibular division, which run from the cochlea and the vestibular apparatus, respectively. The cochlea is a coiled spiral structure (Latin: cochlea = snail shell) which contains receptor cells that are sensitive to vibrations set up by sounds acting on the eardrum. Thus, the cochlear nerve is concerned with hearing.

The vestibular apparatus is a complex system of

liquid filled sacs and tubes which contain receptors sensitive to gravity and acceleration. These receptors, via the cells of the vestibular nerve inform the brain of body position and movement. If the vestibular nerve (or the vestibular apparatus) is destroyed, the sense of balance is impaired. It becomes difficult to maintain an erect posture, especially in the dark or when the eyes are closed.

IX   Glossopharyngeal Nerve

The glossopharyngeal nerve (Greek: glossa = tongue + pharynx) is a mixed nerve carrying taste-sensitive fibres from the tongue, other sensory fibres from the pharynx, plus motor fibres to a muscle in the throat and to the salivary glands.

X   Vagus

The vagus nerve (Latin: vagus = wandering) is a mixed nerve which innervates many of the viscera or internal organs such as the heart, lungs and stomach. By means of sensory vagal fibres the brain is kept informed of the state of these organs and by means of motor vagal fibres it can control their activity. The vagus also contains sensory and motor fibres that run to the pharynx, palate and nearby structures.

XI   Spinal Accessory Nerve

The accessory nerve is a motor nerve carrying fibres that originate in the medulla and others that originate in the spinal cord. These fibres control muscles in the neck and shoulder.

XII   Hypoglossal

The hypoglossal is a motor nerve controlling the muscles of the tongue.

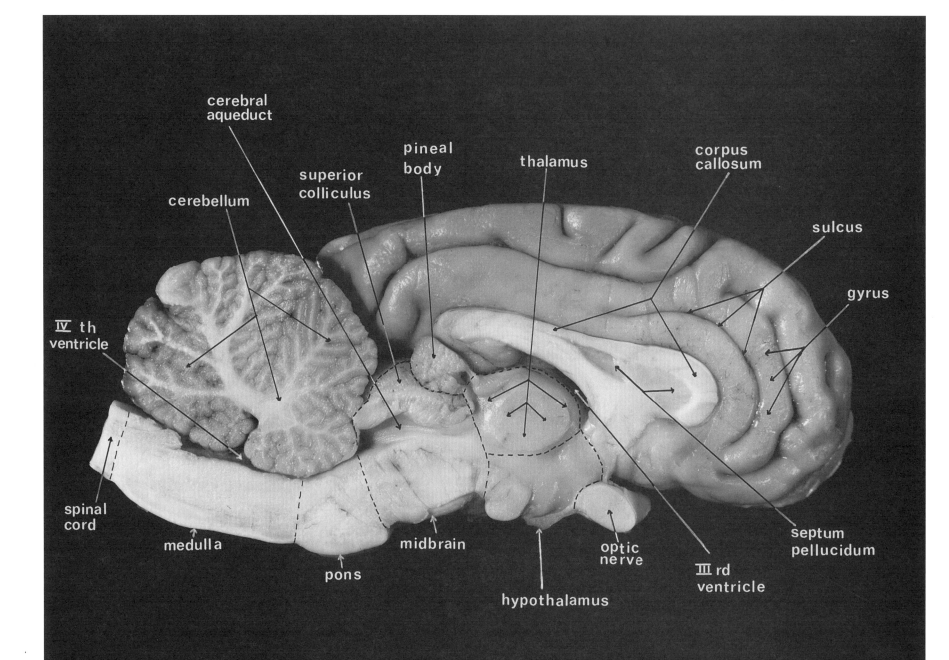

liquid filled sacs and tubes which contain receptors sensitive to gravity and acceleration. These receptors, via the cells of the vestibular nerve inform the brain of body position and movement. If the vestibular nerve (or the vestibular apparatus) is destroyed, the sense of balance is impaired. It becomes difficult to maintain an erect posture, especially in the dark or when the eyes are closed.

IX   Glossopharyngeal Nerve

The glossopharyngeal nerve (Greek: glossa = tongue + pharynx) is a mixed nerve carrying taste-sensitive fibres from the tongue, other sensory fibres from the pharynx, plus motor fibres to a muscle in the throat and to the salivary glands.

X   Vagus

The vagus nerve (Latin: vagus = wandering) is a mixed nerve which innervates many of the viscera or internal organs such as the heart, lungs and stomach. By means of sensory vagal fibres the brain is kept informed of the state of these organs and by means of motor vagal fibres it can control their activity. The vagus also contains sensory and motor fibres that run to the pharynx, palate and nearby structures.

XI   Spinal Accessory Nerve

The accessory nerve is a motor nerve carrying fibres that originate in the medulla and others that originate in the spinal cord. These fibres control muscles in the neck and shoulder.

XII   Hypoglossal

The hypoglossal is a motor nerve controlling the muscles of the tongue.

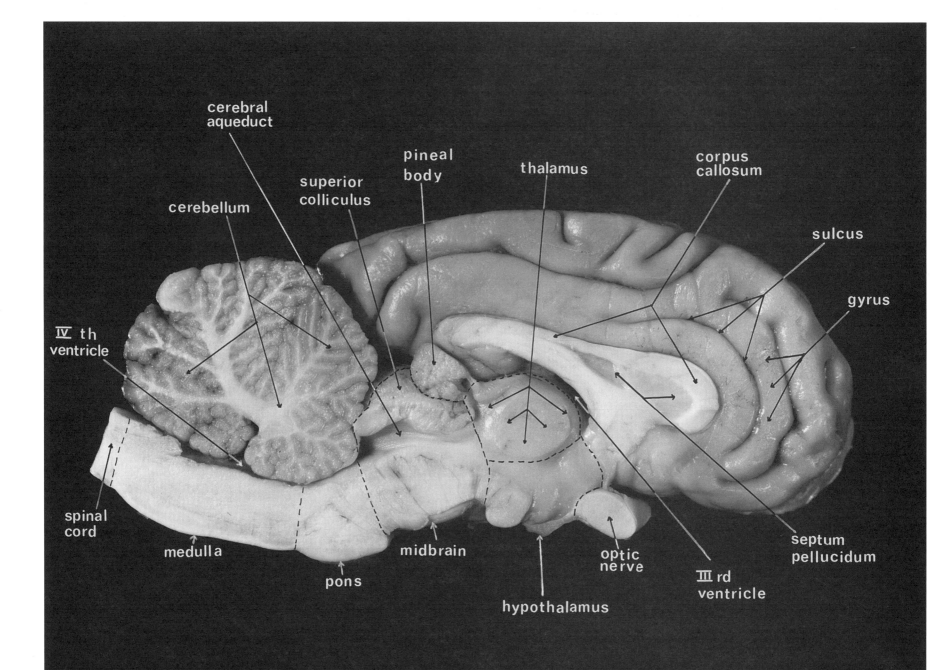

cerebral
aqueduct

superior
colliculus

pineal
body

thalamus

corpus
callosum

cerebellum

sulcus

gyrus

IV th
ventricle

spinal
cord

medulla

pons

midbrain

hypothalamus

optic
nerve

III rd
ventricle

septum
pellucidum

Figure 6. Medial view of a sheep brain.

When the intact sheep brain has been thoroughly examined, cut it into right and left halves to expose the medial surfaces. To do this, place the brain on a table, ventral surface downward. Place a knife with a long thin blade in the medial longitudinal fissure. Then, with a single smooth stroke, cut the brain in half.

Figure 6 shows the main structures visible in a medial view of the sheep brain. Gross divisions of the central nervous system including the spinal cord, medulla, pons, midbrain, thalamus and hypothalamus are demarcated by dotted lines. The thalamus and hypothalamus together are often called the diencephalon. The great mass of tissue lying rostral, dorsal and lateral to the diencephalon constitutes one cerebral hemisphere.

Notice that the brain contains a series of interconnected hollow spaces. These spaces, the brain ventricles, are filled with cerebrospinal fluid during life. They also contain a thin tissue in which many blood vessels are visible. This is the choroid plexus, a tissue which is largely responsible for the formation of the cerebrospinal fluid.

Each cerebral hemisphere contains a separate lateral ventricle which becomes visible when the septum pellucidum is pulled away. Notice that lateral to the septum the lateral wall of the lateral ventricle consists of a large rounded structure. This is the caudate nucleus, so called because it tapers out in a long tail. The roof of the lateral ventricles is the corpus callosum, a system of myelinated and unmyelinated fibres which interconnects areas of the neocortex in one hemisphere with the corresponding areas of the neocortex in the other hemisphere. The lateral ventricles open into the IIIrd ventricle which is a space separating the right and left halves of the hypothalamus and thalamus. The separation is incomplete since the right and left thalami of sheep are connected across the midline by a large mass, the massa intermedia. The IIIrd ventricle communicates with the midbrain. The IVth ventricle is a large space between the cerebellum above and the medulla and pons below. It continues as a long thin tube, the central canal, which runs down the center of the spinal cord.

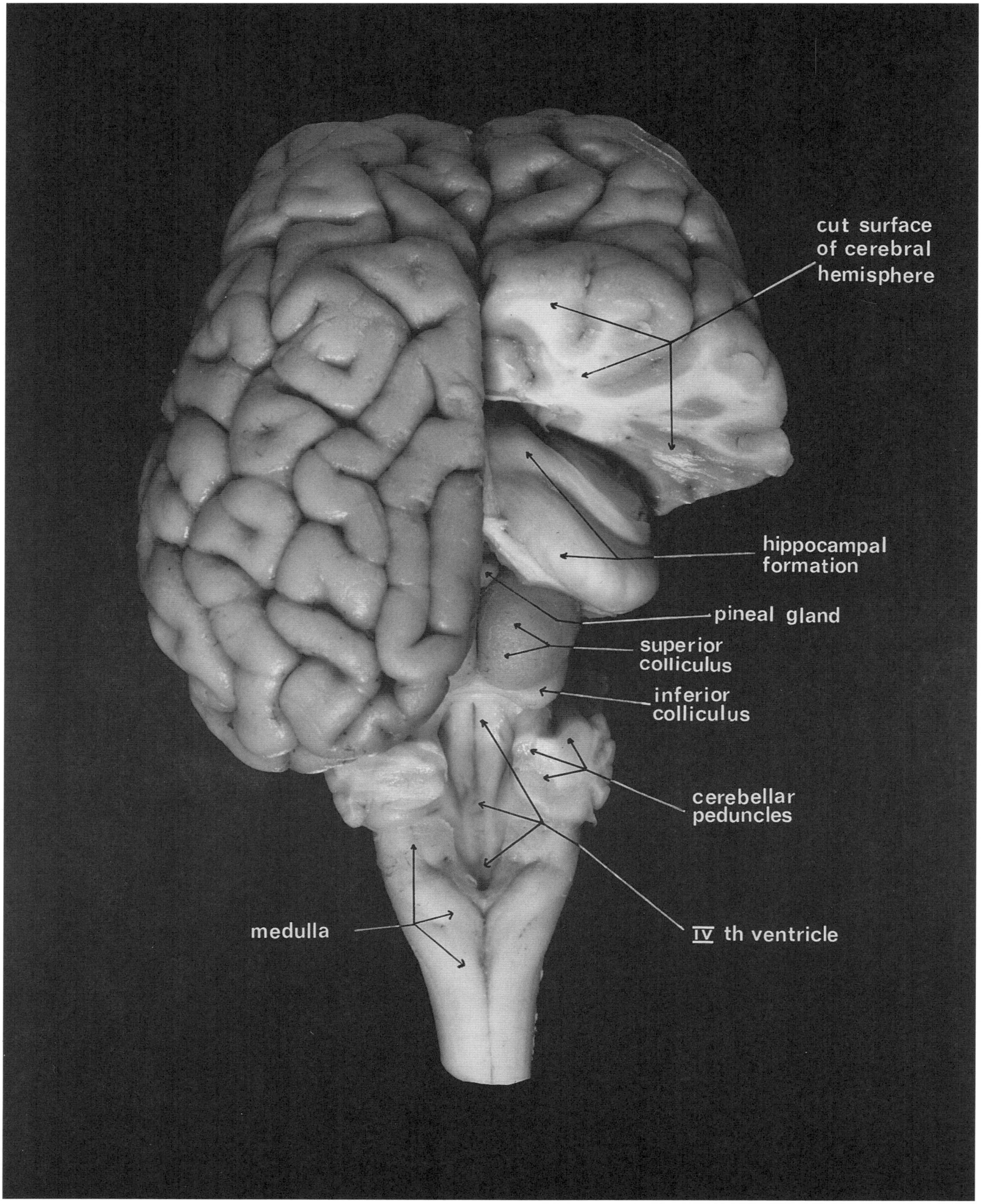

cut surface
of cerebral
hemisphere

hippocampal
formation

pineal gland

superior
colliculus

inferior
colliculus

cerebellar
peduncles

IV th ventricle

medulla

Figure 7. Dissection showing the hippocampal formation and dorsal brainstem.

The dissection shown here was produced by removal of the cerebellum and the caudal half of the right neocortex and corpus callosum. To remove the cerebellum gently pull the caudal end of the medulla ventralward to open the IVth ventricle. The floor of the IVth ventricle is an elongated hollow partly filled by a rounded structure (part of the cerebellum) medial to the laterally placed cerebellar peduncles. These peduncles can be cut through with a scalpel, taking care not to damage the medulla and pons. The cerebellar peduncles contain nerve fibres connecting the cerebellum with the spinal cord, brainstem and thalamus.

The neocortex is best removed by scraping it away with a thin piece of wood. The soft grey matter of the cortex can be removed rapidly, but proceed more cautiously when the deeper white matter is reached. Below the white matter lies the lateral ventricle which can be pulled open to facilitate removal of the remaining overlying neocortex. This will expose the hippocampal formation, a type of cortex shaped somewhat like a ram's horn. Note that the lateral ventricle ends as a pocket not far above the surface of the pyriform lobe and adjacent to the ventral tip of the hippocampal formation.

Removal of the caudal neocortex exposes the superior (rostral) colliculus, the inferior (caudal) colliculus and the pineal gland as well as the hippocampal formation (Latin: colliculus = little mound). The terms superior and inferior are survivors from an old system used to name parts of the body. A "superior" structure is one which has a higher position than an "inferior" structure in a human standing erect.

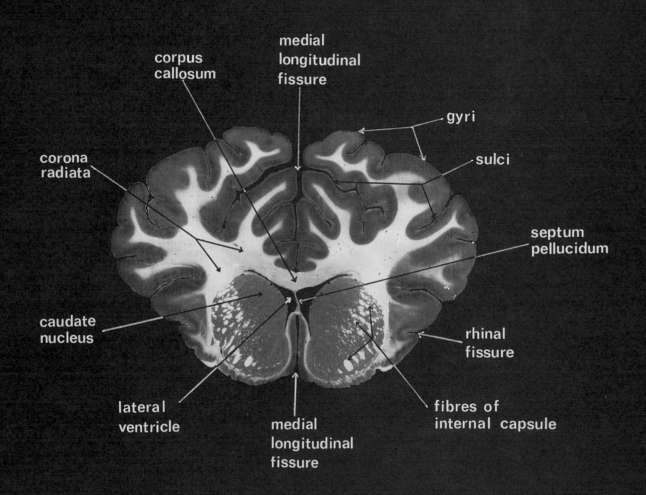

corpus
callosum

medial
longitudinal
fissure

gyri

sulci

corona
radiata

septum
pellucidum

caudate
nucleus

rhinal
fissure

lateral
ventricle

medial
longitudinal
fissure

fibres of
internal capsule

Figure 8. Cross section of the sheep brain at the level of the caudate nucleus.

The photographs in Figures 8, 9 and 10 were prepared from 70 μ thick sections cut from frozen tissue using a device called a microtome (Greek: mikros = small + tome = a cutting). The sections were placed on a glass slide, moistened with a few drops of 1.0% gelatin solution, and used as "negatives" in a photographic enlarger. It is important to keep the sections moist. A solution of gelatin (1.0 gms gelatin powder plus water to make 100 mls of solution) was used for this in preference to water or saline because it has a low surface tension, allowing the sections to lie flat on the glass slide.

Cross sections made through a sheep brain with a knife will not reveal all the details visible in Figures 8 and 9, but the main features can be discerned. To make such a cross section, place the brain on a table, ventral surface downward, and make cuts as shown on the cutting guide on page 24. Cut "A" corresponds to Figure 8 and cut "B" corresponds to Figure 9.

A clear understanding of how the various structures of the brain are placed in relation to one another can be obtained by comparing cross sections with ventral, dorsal, lateral and medial views. It is helpful to cut a brain in sections, examine them, and then reassemble the pieces in their original order.

When examining the cross sections, notice the depth of the cortical sulci and the sharp contrast between the grey tissue of the cortex and the deeper white matter. Part of this white matter consists of myelinated fibres running from the thalamus to the neocortex. As these fibres leave the thalamus they are arranged in thick bundles or in a band referred to as the internal capsule. As the fibres ascend to the neocortex they fan out (radiate) to form the corona radiata. Some of the fibres in the corona radiata and internal capsule originate from cells in the neocortex rather than the thalamus. These fibres may descend to the thalamus (thus creating the possibility of two-way communication between thalamus and cortex) but may also run to other parts of the central nervous system.

The fibres of the corpus callosum interconnect the right and left cerebral hemispheres, particularly the neocortices. The arrangement is such that a cell in a particular location in a gyrus in one hemisphere will send its axon to the corresponding point in the other hemisphere. In this way, the activity of the two hemispheres is kept in step. If the corpus callosum fails to develop normally, or if it is sectioned surgically, the two hemispheres can operate independently to a considerable degree.

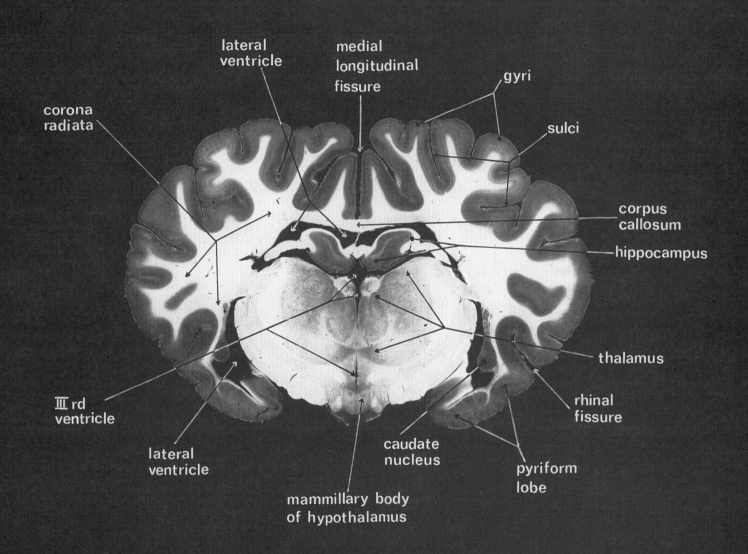

lateral ventricle

medial longitudinal fissure

gyri

corona radiata

sulci

corpus callosum

hippocampus

thalamus

Ⅲ rd ventricle

rhinal fissure

lateral ventricle

caudate nucleus

pyriform lobe

mammillary body of hypothalamus

Figure 9. Cross section of the sheep brain at the level of the thalamus.

In examining a section made at this level note that the hippocampal formation is now visible dorsal to the thalamus, that the caudate nucleus has dwindled to a thin tail and that the entire hemisphere has grown considerably broader than in the section shown in Figure 8. Also note that the lateral ventricle appears in two places in Figure 9. The reason for this is that the ventricle follows a curved "C" shape such that the plane of the cross section intersects it at two points. This can also happen in the case of the hippocampal formation if a cut is made somewhat caudal to the level of Figure 9.

The thalamus is a large structure in the brain which receives input from all the main senses. Different subsections (nuclei) of the thalamus receive information from the eye, the ear, sense organs in the skin and joints as well as inputs from the tongue which signal taste. For the most part, sense organs on the left side of the body send an input to the right side of the thalamus while sense organs on the right side of the body send an input to the left side of the thalamus. Thus, the input is said to be "crossed" or "decussated" (Latin: decussare = to cross in the form of an X). Most of the fibres leaving the thalamus run to the neocortex on the same side of the brain. Some, however, run to the caudate nucleus, hypothalamus and other brain structures.

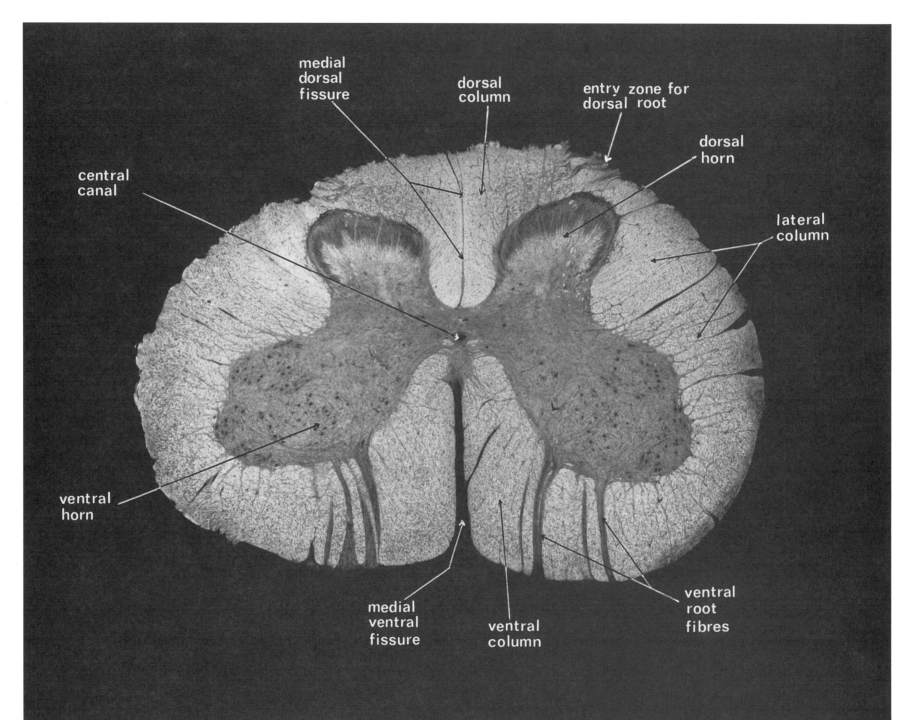

medial
dorsal
fissure

dorsal
column

entry zone for
dorsal root

dorsal
horn

central
canal

lateral
column

ventral
horn

medial
ventral
fissure

ventral
column

ventral
root
fibres

Figure 10. Cross section of the cervical spinal cord of a cow.

This photograph was prepared from a cow spinal cord rather than sheep spinal cord because the larger size makes the procedure easier. Magnification for the cross section of the spinal cord is about 12X actual size. In comparison, magnification for the photographs of the sheep brain is about 2X actual size.

Note that the outside of the spinal cord is a glistening white owing to the presence of large numbers of longitudinally running myelinated nerve fibres. These fibres are regarded as being arranged in three columns (dorsal, lateral and ventral) on each side of the spinal cord. Each of the columns contain both ascending (sensory) fibres running up to the brain and descending (motor) fibres running from the brain to the spinal cord. Still other fibres interconnect different levels of the spinal cord itself.

The interior of the spinal cord contains a "butterfly" of grey matter consisting mainly of cell bodies and fine unmyelinated nerve fibres. This grey matter is subdivided into right and left dorsal horns and right and left ventral horns. Sometimes a small bump on the side of each ventral horn is referred to as the lateral horn.

The center of the spinal cord contains a small tubular space, the central canal, which is connected to the IVth ventricle.

A peripheral nerve connected to the spinal cord contains both sensory and motor fibres. Near the cord the nerve divides in a "Y" shape. The dorsal arm of the Y (called the dorsal root) contains only sensory fibres and is attached to the cord adjacent to the dorsal horn. The ventral root contains only motor fibres and is attached to the cord adjacent to the ventral horn. Thus, sensory fibres coming in from the skin or the muscles, for example, enter the dorsal horn. At some point they may make synaptic contact with other neurons which run rostrally to the brain, or they may make contact directly with the ventral horn cells. The ventral horn cells (visible as dark granules in the ventral horn in Figure 10) have axons that run out in the ventral roots to the muscles. Activity in these cells causes the muscles to contract. It is therefore possible for a sensory stimulus to produce a motor response (movement) via a chain of only two neurons separated by a single set of synapses. An example of a situation where this actually happens is the sudden jerk or kick of the lower leg which can be elicited in a human by tapping sharply on the patellar tendon just below the knee cap. This should be done while the subject sits on a bench or table with the lower part of the leg hanging freely. If the knee jerk is weak or absent its amplitude can usually be increased (in a normal subject) by tensing muscles elsewhere in the body (e.g. clenching the fists or the teeth).

Simple sensori-motor reactions, such as the knee jerk, are often called reflexes. The knee jerk is often said to be a monosynaptic reflex since its occurrence is dependent on only one synaptic junction. More complex reflexes are referred to as disynaptic, trisynaptic or polysynaptic.

In terms of the activity of the leg muscles, a voluntary kick of the lower leg may be identical to a reflex kick of the same leg. However, the neural circuits responsible for the two behaviors are quite different. A reflex can occur as a result of activity in as few as two neurons but a voluntary movement occurs as a result of complex patterns of activity involving large areas of the brain. This activity results in nerve impulses which descend from the brain to activate the spinal neurons.

Cutting guide for Figures 8 and 9.

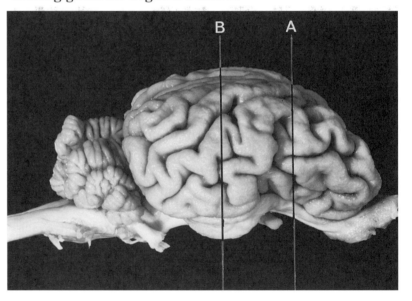